Dedicated: To all of the people in the nursing field that I have met and grown to like and love. It takes the whole team to make it work. From the physical therapist to even some of the doctors.

Tamiko B.,Victoria T. ,Mazie B., Melaine J., Colleen M., Jennifer R. Dr. Briles., Dr. Bown,Toya H., Lakesha G.,Kenitra H., Fadizso J.,Victoria G.,Monica R., Rosalba,Maria,Austin V,Mitzy,Angie, Sarah, Laquinta,Ciara Rebecca, Rebecca D. and Christy D. Dalina,Edith,Elaun,Elma,Fontera, Francesca,Jessica D.,Kathy, Karen,Kamelaya,Lencha,Linda,Mae, Melissa G., Michael, Tina S.,Shanquel,Sonia D., Robert"Skip",Whitney,Pamela from Sarasota,Pam From Tampa,Lanaidra S.,CarlineM.,LuLuB.,Marlene,Albert,Suz anne,Susan M.,Suesan,Cindy,Michelle C., Everyone at St. Josephs,Terry I miss you.Melissa P.,Jessica, Amanda you are going to kick ass as a nurse you beautiful porcelain red headed doll.

Mary my Philippine queen you're awesome and I appreciate you.
Arda your retirement will suit you.
Teressa less stress to come. Iresenia get your own business on the internet and let someone else handle the customers.Tiffany take your medicine after the baby is born take it.
Jessica you're an awesome person,wife,mother and director of nursing.
I love you Adrienne you will always have Jamaica. Shelley you are the epitome of beauty and grace and you are an awesome boss. Yes Barbara when I saw you snap over a piece of paper I was scared and I knew then but you will be great at anything you choose. Ron you have passed on allot of wisdom thank you. Lottie keep it real you beautiful queen. Quanda and her husband Manny Alliseandrea you are beautiful in every way,I pray you get what you want in every way. My girl Katie remember your health before wealth.

The beautiful blonde headed woman that
enters the room and fills it with grace and
poetry my dear Jena your time is coming.

I think you're a little hyper but I don't
hate you Michelle. Love you always
Kisha and although I do love myself she
just happens to have the same name.
Nichole, My other Nikki Nicole I miss
our nights of fun but I will always
treasure them. Terrance M. I will never
look at a kitchen,bathroom,or conference
room the same in a nursing home and I
forgot our breaks in the car yummy.
My beautiful sister Spring the future
Doctor former Nursing Assistant don't
give up.

The friendships I have had over the years
I will always cherish because even
though people say; I am not here to make
friends I am here to work. That never
seemed to apply to me. Please forgive me
if I didn't mention you, but hell it's been
twenty years.

The Dark Side of Nursing

People think of nursing often in categories: Doctors, Registered Nurses, License Nurses, Physical Therapist and Certified Nursing Assistant. Depending on who you ask they all provide a valuable role in the care and recovery of patients.

Well you are putting your loved one in a nursing home or hospital. You pay allot of money for this five star treatment and you expect that service.
As well as you should, but remember the ones running the show is getting that money, and we are not.

"Truth "the worst nursing homes stay open because the state needs to put the poor people somewhere. So as long as there alive and have no family or resources.

That little funding that they pretend to provide is kickback for allowing them to stay in business "slum lords to the fifth power" and the state to say we put your tax dollars and funding to good use.

Nursing use to be a special profession where, people cared and this is the one place where caring should be the top priority, after all we are caregivers.

In the last twenty years it has become a money racket. Full of uncaring want to be paid above the minimum wage no people skills people.

They don't care anymore it's how much money we can make and try not to kill anyone today. The nursing field hasn't developed characteristics of Publix when it comes to customer service. However that being said people are often much nicer when the buying food, rich or poor we all want to eat.

It shouldn't matter where you come from or how much money you have, who your family is, but it does in the mind of people that are still are once was affluent. It should have no baring in the kind of care you receive or how they receive it.

Family likes to remind you that they pay your salary and we are the Wellingtons if we say jump you ask how high. The bosses that are there from 9-5 like to promote this behavior after all it's their money on the line.

People even on their dying bed want to throw their weight around and their prestige. Their families that feel guilty sometimes or just use to giving them whatever they want, and want us to do the same.

They are sometimes rude and mean to the people you are leaving them with and you want them to do their damn job, just do it and smile and do it now. Then you leave, You can't be there 24/7 so what do you think happens when you leave.

Do you really want to know?

I have worked in nursing twenty two years being a Certified Nursing Assistant and I am very proud of that. Anyone else that wants to go further I encourage them, go as far as you can. It is stressful humbling ,hard work and it use to be rewarding.

If you live in the Florida and are African American, Haitian, Jamaican or Chinese you can become LPN if you take the test more the once. If you want to be a RN they fail you sight unseen, whatever you put on the application other than white you fail.

No matter where you live in Florida the men and woman have to take extreme measures in order to pass the test and they take it more than once at four to eight hundred a pop and two thousand dollars or more each time they have to take it again the refresher course.

People do not view you as a real nurse if you're not a RN.

It does not matter or well it shouldn't matter what level you are, from janitor to Doctor everyone should be valued. Since there not always valued monetarily or treated with no respect you get substandard care. Just because we chose this profession does not mean, we chose what came next. Remember it was not always like this.

Before lawsuit happy people on both sides of the spectrum, we had people that actually cared and they are still out there, it is just very few.

I know people from the
Philipines,Tawain,Canada,Jamaica,Haiti,
Puerto Rico and all over these United
States that went into this field with a
good heart and the woes of the field
either broke them or left them wondering
why they ever done this.

We are human too, we have our breaking
points, most people in nursing have some
psych issues after three to five years.
We've learned how to smile and hate at
the same time, learning how to say ok no
problem, while visualizing running you
over with a car.

These are truths as only I can tell them
you have not seen what I have seen. Now
when it comes to poor nursing homes. It
is true you get what you pay for,
understaffed over worked people, that no
longer care.

The place reeks of urine as soon as you
walk in, you can smell the bed sores from
a mile away. The stench of unclean
bodies feel the air.

Have you heard this before? We here at nursing rehab take great pleasure in providing quality care for your loved ones. We are a five star facility, which gives you choices in the food and activities you seek for your love ones.

We are all about the quality of care for the extended or short life of your love one.

All bullshit that is the Admissions department they are like used car sells men. They are told to close the deal and read the people and tell them exactly what they want to hear.

No matter what, when you take a tour they show you the best part of the facility. It is usually during the week and in the day time where they can make interference where they have to.

When it is time the counselor comes out to meet with you and your family. To close the deal they find out how much money and assets you have. Do they need to tell the family it is best if we take care of the all the paper work to ensure you get the best possible care.

Translation we drain every possible resource Medicaid, Medicare your personal insurance and when it runs out they kick you out.

All of sudden you get sick and they have to send you out. You try to return and they do not have a bed for you, you are told it is full. What has happened is simple your insurance can not pay for it anymore.
They will legally screw you. If you have no money or family you are as good as dead.

Why do you think you come into the nursing home one week and the next week they are dead. I did not realize they were that sick they need the bed for someone that can pay.

If you take prescription Benadryl and don't eat for a week you die. Ask what the medications is for and what it is. It doesn't matter, the standard answer this is what the doctor ordered and this the best plan of action that was prescribed.

You don't like it talk to the Doctor who is unavailable until it is too late. Scream negligence until the cows come home if you are poor or otherwise. You have to prove it. C.Y.A. is a term we use in nursing cover your own ass. They stress documentation over care, you can't prove what you say or what you see.

What's in black in white can be challenged or explained away. When you visit your family if you care do not be predictable if they know you're coming and what days and time you are coming. The bells and whistles are on until you leave.

The resident can be wonderful and the family a nightmare. Well no resident no nightmares. You don't believe me. They just lost their balance, they fell out of bed I just transferred them from the shower to the chair and they just fell. Yes were giving them something for the pain.

They just had a heart attack out of the blue. Did you know if you shoot someone with insulin between their toes or the inside of their fingers or where the genital area is too much insulin gives you a heart attack.

Be aware and be nice or fake it. It can happen in all nursing homes but if, your low on the totem poll, you are virtually invisible. Your invisible to the state and the city also to the officials lawyers cost money.

The state is overwhelmed and the can only work on the case or an allegation for a short time. You can be wrapped up in paperwork for a long time and at the end of it all you are is appeased.

Remember the worst nursing homes can have a five star rating. It does not have to be the whole nursing home. This is why nursing rehabilitation units where invented. It is usually the rehab unit that gets the five stars.

Therefore legally the facility can call themselves a five star facility. This is not hotel or restaurant, but because our minds are wired a certain way and they can trick you with what you think you know. Psychologist and marketing analysts invent the language of nursing.

It is subsequent programming, How can I help you? Can I do anything to make you comfortable? I apologize that, that occurred we will do our very best to ensure it doesn't happen again.

We will do our very best to get to the bottom of this be assured we are taking all the necessary precautions. If you are a problem or become one they will beyond a shadow of a doubt get rid of you legally.

There are many gray areas of nursing , food ,cleanliness,supplies,infestations. You or your insurance pays three hundred or more a day for a room usually you are sharing with another person.

Even in the most expensive nursing homes, let's face it more people more money. I usually pay four hundred dollars a week for a cruise, I get the best food variety and all I can eat or drink and entertainment.

For what you pay you should have chefs making your food everyday now in some of nicer nursing homes they do. However this is something you have paid into usually which is transitional care.

You buy into the community, stay in the high rise independent living, then and if you get to where you can't take care of yourself then you have already paid into the nursing home.

It is a few of these that is held for the very elite and again even they are flawed but I will get into that later.

For the people that work in the kitchen they usually get paid minimum wage up to nine dollars an hour they are not chefs. They are usually following a step by step all around town menu.

What the kids have for lunch and breakfast in school that is usually what they are having. It is mandated by the state hence forth legal in all of the United States.

A low sodium, low concentrated sweets diet nothing individualized really, you may have a few choices if you don't like the main meal. Of sandwich or sandwich maybe a fruit plate, eggs and toast every day with a side of hot or cold cereal.

If the resident have been there more than a week they already know what their having and it's not always good. If their incoherent they might not care or incapacitated.

That is not the point the best possible care should mean the best possible meals as well. It doesn't happen, it is sad but true.

When choosing a nursing home for your loved ones. It shouldn't be the hospital recommendations or someone visiting you patrolling for your money.

You should choose a nursing home like you choose your house. Location and great care most nursing homes have a twenty four hour policy and they have codes to get into the building.

Don't go just in the day time, go and pop up in the evening, you really want to know about the nursing home and be told the absolute truth become friends with a Nursing assistant or janitor. Legally we cannot say the names, but we can damn sure pose a hypothetical.

A staged meeting oppose to a meeting they set up and come more than one day. What do I mean by stage meeting texting

Kisha and saying lets have lunch and showing up and getting lost looking for her.

If they have security they will page the person if their there and you won't get pass the front entrance.

Don't fret there is a way around this as well, donate anything to the residents and staff. Just say for one day you want to volunteer and do bingo. You don't get a true since of a place unless your there. This may seem extreme but so is bad food and death.

They lie to us as well, they say you are doing Gods work if you choose this profession there is nothing more rewarding. The first couple of years you believe this lie or you want to believe it.

No matter if you're a registered nurse, licensed nurse or certified nursing assistant you are not just doing the job you went to school for or was trained for.

You have to become adaptable to your surroundings and each given situation. You become tactical and emotionally configured.

Anger should not be shown or given, hand gestures should be no part of your overall demeanor, facial expressions should be one and one only or kept to minimum eyebrows should never be raised and your voice needs to be kept a certain tone and pitch.

For this alone I should be getting paid more money.

I understand the downsizing of a company they want more bang for the buck. Hire less people and give the ones we have three jobs that way we save money at the expense of the people that need to feed their families. They either do it or they find some one that will. You are responsible for getting nine grown people dress and clean.

You are responsible for making sure they are fed, showered, shaved and their family also kept happy. Making sure they go to activities or physical therapy. It can be overwhelming nine or more personalities that you are caring for plus their family and the five personalities you are suppressing.

The suffering is the people, if a post office worker gets stressed and kills or the stock broker that killed himself because he lost money. What do you think happens to verbally abused, underappreciated and underpaid people in nursing.

We are dealing with people not product on an assembly line, but that is the way the company treats them move them in ship them out. They die get the bed full no empty beds allowed, every bed empty is money loss. To the big companies it is business as usual some of them never even step foot into a nursing home.

There bottom line is money and how much they can get of it. They allocate money for law suits and mishaps. The worst nursing homes makes three million dollars a month so if they have more than one nursing home and they usually do.

They look at how they can keep their cost down no injuries, no lawsuits and less people more work.

I am going to tell you how this works and this is really how your money is being spent. Also what goes on behind the scenes. How the state plays the role on how the facility is ran, from the supplies to the front door. How rich people and their nursing homes get away with racism and murder.

How they get away with this on paper? Why there is no such thing as not enough help? How they are never under staffed on paper. In nursing that is all that matters.

Located in the front of every facility is a record or a book located somewhere visible. That of course people don't usually look at. It tells you how many people that are on staff, and also tells you there facility rating. Located right above that is usually how much they charge per day.

This rate is just the basics food and shelter, for every service required or recommended by the doctor is an extra cost. If you need to be administered medicine, if you need physical therapy or occupational therapy and if you need speech therapy.

They even charge for soap and for the most part crappy food.

All additional cost long term care verses, short term care, young verses old, whether you are in your right mind or not is all a part of how much they get and how fast they get it.

The doctors that treat the patients has a vested interest in the nursing homes, then the trusted doctor recommends the nursing home he frequents. He informs the patient to speak the admissions coordinator. This happens so fast that you don't even remember if you really need rehab or not.

Money is the under tone if you think it is not don't be fooled. Yes it varies are there good nursing homes, no not really just one is better than the other and like our President you have to choose the lesser of the evils. I know this is not an easy decision and it can be a stressful one.

However if I am old or dying slowly I would like to know I still have choices, I would like to know I could still have breyers ice cream or the taste wasn't taken out of my food when I'm ninety.

Damn it, don't give me tasteless food and don't leave me for twelve hours in a wet diaper. Don't make me pee on myself and forget about me.

Please don't hurt me because I can no longer speak. Please turn on the television because all of my children are dead and everyone I know dead. Just sounds of other people's voices is keeping me connected.

To help me to understand I am alive and I pray this isn't hell.

I didn't make you angry don't yell at me. I didn't mean to drool please clean my face. Don't leave me without my hair done. I was once beautiful and independent.

Please don't forget I am a person and not a paycheck!!!!!!!

All nursing homes are not created equal, some of them use pads to make sure the bed doesn't get wet and the patient is not uncomfortable and some of them don't.

At night to save cost for 11-7 they don't use briefs which are adult diapers. This is also the shift that has less help because they should be sleeping so you get twenty patients all legal.

As long as they prove, they have enough nursing assistants in the building it doesn't matter what they are doing or even if they are on that particular unit. It just matters how many there are divided by the amount of residents.

So they can count the nursing assistants and nurses from the day before to make it look like they have enough staff for the whole week.

This is usually the job of the director of Nursing but she can blame the person that makes less money than her that she hired as staffing coordinator if shit hits the fan. By shit I mean disgruntle family members and the state.

What about evaluations that are mandated by the state? What about them? The state comes once a year to do a survey and if no one has complaints or calls the state they don't come back. All of the nursing homes make sure they are doing their very best. The best food, more help on the floor, everybody pitching in from Head to tail.

Isn't it supposed to be a surprise? Yes, but people develop friendships over time and if one nursing home is getting visited by the state then the others in that immediate area know they are within their window.

Again I am a firm believer if you do things right all year long you don't have to worry about it.

But who am I kidding this in nursing.

What you have in your bank account and what you know matters.

Don't assume anything when it comes to nursing. Don't assume people give a damn about your wellbeing just because they are in the healthcare field. It's like those old cartoons you are a barely breathing, continuous care dollar sign.

It is unfortunate that it is true even at the end of your life money matters. You pay more you usually get more. There are some nursing homes that don't except people of color. Of course in the south even the nursing homes are segregated.

When you are both poor however that is not an issue.

The doctors coordinate with nurses and admissions. You have to check off race without thinking about it and you also have to check off your financial capability which predetermines your fate.

Usually everyone is so connected and skillful at what they do the chain and flow of money never stops. Nursing homes should not be a scary place but sometimes it is and it is becoming worse.

When you put profit before people it is never a good scenario. The competition for this is fierce, everyone is trying hard to keep the beds full, thus keeping their bank accounts full.

I know what you're thinking, this is also how they pay you. I have never had a problem finding a job unless I was hurt. Nursing is twenty four hour job and I have been doing it for twenty years.

There are agencies to work for, private duty, the hospital it is so many facets of nursing you are never without the means of work.

It is the process and bureaucracy that I am oppose to. How people on both ends are getting taking advantage of patients and workers.

You are in a twenty four hour facility and somehow an agency convinces you, you need twenty four hour care on top of your stay at the nursing home to make sure you are properly maintained.

What? Why? Fear and guilt are the weapons of choice and because of this many people are willing victims.

Make no mistake they know this and they use these very means to take your money. I have seen it with my own eyes. People crying because they have to give up their assets. Homes they have been in for years their 401ks and their life savings and they are convinced to.

The nursing home raises the prices and criteria every year. Social Security is not a viable sustainable source of income so they are robbed, and forced into a lifestyle where it use to be 1200 or more square feet to 200 still paying the full amount and sharing a room with a total stranger.

In twenty years you can imagine that I have visited over a hundred homes and over fifty nursing homes as a Certified Nursing Assistant and a Private Duty aide I am sure it is allot more but I lost count but I could never erase what I have experienced and seen.

It is not all horrible but I see headed there. Yes there are lawyers that fight wrongful death suits and elderly abuse cases. Remember in nursing it is all about verbiage and documentation. Did it really happen the way you saw or did you hear what you think you heard.

So these are my untold stories just a few, but even these should inform you and educate you from the first to the last.

When I first started in the nursing field I had a rude awakening. I got hit, spit on, called nigger , feces and pee throw at me sexually assaulted and verbally abused. I was told each time that they are our means of living and you can put on file, but you cannot call the police or make a police report this is a part of nursing.

If you are to abuse a resident however there is a hotline. Nothing however put in place to help the people take care of them. For a long time I couldn't understand this logic and I still don't . This is just how it is and if you don't want to work there is the door.

What are you suppose to do your making above minimum wage and you're a single mother with three mouths to feed. You do what all good mothers do you suck it up and make the best of it.

This is where the multiple personalities start to develop but you don't even realize it.

I was proud of my work I worked hard and long hours. Before anyone gave us Hoyer lifts to pick up the patients, we were expected to do this. The young ladies before me didn't even have the privilege of gloves so I considered myself lucky.

I worked at my first nursing home at twenty three it was an all African American Staff and Administration all of the residents as well.

They couldn't afford other nursing homes so I thought it was pretty cool. It was a bit to get use to but I didn't know any better it was my first job in nursing. I didn't know I was getting slave wages and doing allot work.

I use to hear those residents cries in my sleep, I use to wake up in the middle of the night to go check on them. It was mentally taxing. People weren't put to bed sometimes to twelve o'clock in the morning or later then it was up five o'clock for breakfast. I worked while my children were in daycare in the morning.

If you are in nursing the best hours to work is on the weekend or eleven to seven twelve hour shifts and sixteen hour shifts. This is how you can make more money and have a job during the week, so you can make a decent life for your family even if you are a nurse you usually have two and three jobs to just be comfortable.

Well I know what you are thinking, so what most Americans have two and three jobs , what's the big deal. No sleep, taking care of children, not eating properly may work for delivering mail, but it doesn't work when dealing with people.

Your family and social life suffers it is the ultimate trickle down affect. I am not telling you what I think I am telling you what I know. Nurse comes in not even changed from her other job, she is giving report because they have to. She is not really paying attention she is tire but you have a body there.

She is giving her medicine to all the residents and at the end of the night she realizes that she hasn't checked on the patient all night and neither has the c.n.a because she is sleep somewhere tired from her other job.

They get in there the resident is dead probably has been for hours. You have to call 911 anyway and rigamortis has set in. Remember back then it was just elderly people sixty to eighty residents, three c.n.a.s and one nurse.

So you put them in hot water to raise
their body temperature,
Change their clothes then call 911 when
their body temperature is past 99.9
degrees. Wrap them in blankets , poor
scolding hot water down their throat, put
in the documentation that you checked on
them every two hours.

They already old so them dying just is a
part of life. I saw it and didn't think
anything of it I just thought how
amazingly thorough they were.

It happened allot and if you cannot move
or speak , you really have a short life
span it is harsh but true. You may leave
that day and come back to this individual
what happened to Miss Ashton. She
rolled herself outside and fell out of the
chair she is in the hospital.

Well first of all she was contracted how
could she do that. I don't know, I didn't
see it but that is what they said.

Assumption doesn't work with the cops and damn sure doesn't transpire into nursing, you can suspect all you want but if you didn't see it, it didn't happen. When your heart is in it you want to try to help them all but the sad fact is you can't. Not mentally or physically only thing that is twenty four hours is God really.

There was the patient let's call her Ms. Essie that every day at about five o'clock she would relive her father raping her. She would scream it great detail everyday reliving it as if it was happening now. What do you do?

That kind of torment you can't train for. I use to whisper in her ear he is dead we killed him sister. Every day I whispered in her ear something to that effect but nothing ever worked.

She would still relive that horrible day over and over again until she died. That Alzheimer's and dementia is a cruel disease. That even in our last days we cannot escape from our most horrible memories. On the other hand it can also just replay a good memory every day I guess it is solace in that.

The first thing they tell you in nursing is to keep it professional. Don't become attached or personal. Stay on a last name basis. Well again that is good on paper but how do you do that in real life. You see and take care of them every day, you are not a robot. They say this is to help with the process of nursing.

Well how stupid is that. Miss Bell would greet me every day she couldn't remember what day it was and sometimes she wouldn't remember her kids names. I came in at three everyday if I was late she let me know a minute loss is money lost.

I know I will do better tomorrow. I would talk to her about various things and she would gossip as old ladies do about what went on during the day.

Well the state comes in and ask questions to the residents that they think might give the most truthful answers. She was ninety and as sharp as she could be. The state was coming in the next day because they got a call.

The longer their there, the more stuff they may find out. So no nursing home wants them there longer than they have to be.

I came in the next day as usual I didn't see Miss Bell. I thought she just had a bad day and forgot so I started my shift. I still didn't see her. A couple of hours went by I went to go look for her.

Anybody that has been in nursing when they see an empty bed with no sheets on it know what happened.

My heart sunk and I screamed where is
she, she wasn't sick! The nurse came to
me sometimes these things just happen
all of sudden it is a part of life.

Fuck you, liar you killed her all of you
are going to hell.

Needless to say you can't say that and
keep your job. I was so worried they
could fire me but they can't keep me
from coming up there. Well it turns out
they could.

Those people with their idiosyncrasies
who is going to take care of them. Mrs.
Johnson doesn't like it when people just
pull things over her head, she say you're
not skinning a cat be gentle. Mr. Shannon
who is going to tell him, he is still
handsome and his chair is his new normal
that are plenty reasons to live let's find
one today. Who is going to brush the hair
out of Mrs. Erma eyes because she hates
it there. I cried for days.

I said I am not going to another nursing home. So I worked for someone else for a while but it was not as gratifying. So I tried another nursing home this was a little more upscale. I thought this will be great I am an optimistic so one bad horrendous experience shouldn't keep me away from what I love.

I love people let's do this Kisha we can do this. Whatever happens we will overcome and get through it. It was different and they had enough help the food was great.

Here we go it didn't last long until I saw crazy things happening. Skillful and perfecting foolery is the worst kind.

People that have been in the business for a long time know what to do. They know what is to be expected and what not to do. The difference is their level of compassion and what motivates them.

People that open up nursing homes or agencies because of their loved ones is usually the better place to put them. They are doing it with the right motives and heart. It is only when bureaucracy gets in the middle or in the way is when these ideas are tested or shaken.

There was locked unit in this facility where it seemed to be hidden. That wasn't unusual allot of nursing homes have these. This is where they keep the people that are exit seeking or combative. It's a safety precaution for the other residents as well as themselves.

You had to sign a bunch of papers to even work on this particular unit. Well I got a chance to work on the unit and once you are on the unit, you're there the door locks behind you only one way in and one out. To go on your break was a mini vacation.

This unit was not a regular locked unit, it was people being drugged so they can be maintained. They looked like zombies. It was horrific all lined up for breakfast, lunch and dinner. Everyone on the same diet. Routine care for everyone, none of them spoke just murmured.

When the state would come they never came in this unit and I wondered why. I had to boldness to ask one day a fellow employee. She said why would the state inspect a closet they don't know this exist and if you tell anyone, you are fired.

Anonymous tip they know someone there that handles the phone calls. It has been like this for ten years, they said you cannot inspect what you have no idea about.

These are the unmentionables the ones that the family doesn't visit anymore, the ones the nursing home wants to hide so they don't mess up their reputation.

Why do you think there is no windows she said and we get paid five dollars an hour more to work back here.

I picked up extra shifts and wanted to know if what she was telling me was true. I asked a couple of other people and it was true. Others called them the hidden.

So now I have another moral dilemma are these people that dangerous and they are doing the right thing. Is it something much bigger they are doing the wrong thing and I was being given "I better " hush money.

To a single mother money was a great thing no struggling. So I stayed there for a while the money was great. Then it happened. My head got in the way of my pocket book.

This beautiful lady was brought in, and she had dementia and early onset of Alzheimer's. They said she was always trying to leave. I talked to her for a couple of days because she wasn't a zombie.

She said I want to leave, I just redirected her as I was told to do. She told me how she missed her family and how they put her in here and don't even come and see me.

Well one day someone came to see her, and they took her out of the unit for a day, I thought how nice for her and then she came back sobbing. I told her it is going to be ok Luann and she looked up at me and said bye it was great to have known you.

Ok I said you are not trying to kill yourself are you, no she said but my legal guardian was here with the counselor and they sentenced me to death. They can't sentenced you to death this is not a jail.

Look around she said these people are trapped in their own bodies it is a living hell.

The worst kind of jail when you wake up every day in this body and mind that has turned against you. Trapped but you can't voice your opinions, hurt but you don't know how to communicate that, crying and no tears to speak of.

I feel me slipping away and I can't catch her. When I look in the mirror I don't recognize her. My guardian consented to whatever medicine would be helpful to me.

After a couple of days I saw it too, her slipping away and now like the rest of them a zombie.

How do you fight this legal injustice, to die in dignity should be a right. Not taken away by those you trust and are supposed to care about you.

People that are ignorant to what drugs can do to you, trusting a doctor and his opinion without a second opinion or research.

It should be criminal but it isn't. However it is sad and almost hopeless. I want to do something, but I just don't know what to do or how to go about it.

I called the cops they are not trained in nursing. I told them people are being held against their will in the closet. They couldn't find it , the facility said one of the residents must of called and said sorry and sent them on their way. I called the fire department, the ambulances no one could find it.

A few weeks passed by and I finally got enough nerve to bring someone there. I brought them and said look all the person from the state said, was they see a clean well maintained facility and the people were getting well cared for.

No I told her they make them into
zombies, they weren't like this before
they came here. She put her hand on my
shoulders and said this is the nature of the
disease don't waste our resources again
on nonsense unless there is abuse or
neglect and I don't see any of that here. If
you can't handle this maybe this is the
wrong field for you.

You don't understand I told her this place
is hidden from the world, you need to
grow up she said. Well maybe she was
right I am crazy and this is normal. Then
I looked over at Luann and I chose to
believe my lying eyes. I tried, I failed, I
quit.

Well I chose to do something different I
went to join an agency and do private
care. One on one surely this is better and
less stressful.

What you have to understand is any state people are retiring. Also that all of these services exist in all over the world. In the sunshine state where they often retire and have the most money to do so.

Here is where the problem lies. People

are getting charged for services they don't need, they will probably never get use of allot of things the use to do. In order to get the money out of the families these vultures prey on the families love, fear and hope.

There is always a chance that people will get better and I believe in miracles but some are so farfetched there is no return on them.

Yes they have drugs that help with memory and behavioral issues. The scientist say that they can't really find out if have Alzheimer's until you die. I know you're thinking what everyone says, What? That's messed up it's too late then.

Yes it is but if it runs in your family you can often try to prepare for this outcome. Change in your diet and how you eat to improve your chances, in not getting the disease or prolonging it.

Educate yourselves and stay involved as much as possible.

Now that I have finished that rant let me proceed in telling you about the agency and my experience with them. First of all what they charge the families is a fraction of what the workers get. It still can be a ridiculous amount of money.

I'm with someone and their spouse, you are taking care of just one of them supposedly, you always, always wind up taking care of them both always.

The agencies they pimp you out legally. They tell the families that when the aide gets here she or he will take care of all your needs.

So the families have been led to believe they get a three for one a maid, a caregiver and a cook. It is not their fault they are led to believe this by the agency, that private duty means your slave for the day.

I took care of gentlemen and his wife, where the only thing they wanted me to do was to be on standby. He had a fall previously and he got around well as well as the wife. The children that lived out of state was told that it was unsafe for him to be alone and they couldn't get down for a month.

Well in a months' time that is allot of money and again fear and guilt will convince the inconvincible. To get something they really don't need for their loved ones.

I was there doing almost absolutely nothing but waiting for twelve hours sometimes fourteen. Now I'm not going to lie it felt good to sit down and do nothing for a change.

My damn conscious again, however saw five people at a time coming there and all of them are getting paid.

There is an upfront fee then they bill them by the month or biweekly. How do I know when people get angry that you're in their house they begin to get a little chatty.

They have to have a nurse come in every week. They have to be evaluated by a physical therapist and possibly get physical therapy so they can get back to their best possible life.

Well okay that sounds great but they are sometimes ninety and above they are living their best possible life if they are eating, drinking and thinking on their own.

They are not all of sudden going to run a 5k just because they may have done it twenty years ago. Their bones are not going all of sudden get straight and they are not going to be lifting a 100lbs.

Some of these things are unnecessary but if you don't know otherwise you take it as truth. Everyone for the most part wants the best for the family. Especially as they get older or has a sudden injury or illness.

Around the clock care is not what this couple needed maybe somebody in the afternoon and someone at night to help put him to bed at night. He was sharp ninety but sharp his wife was forgetful and she was a little younger than him but still able to mask it a little.

Just a few hours not twenty four hours. You have to be proactive don't just take somebody's word for it that just may have the wallets best interest and not yours. Remember we are trained to lie to you, it's called customer service.

Now none of it is easy work whether it's a nursing home or their house it is still their home. It is easy to dismiss some ones needs sometimes when we don't share a personal connection with them.

We should not lose our humanity and forget that we are taking care of people. We especially should not be taking advantage of them whether they have money to spend or not. Some people want you to just do whatever and spend their money and they are aware and don't care.

It is very hard to watch people die over and over again. It is also hard to see someone in pain and they are living with that day in and day out. Their only relief it seems to be death.

We live and learn on this journey called life and we can choose to do something about what we see or do what everyone else does.

When you are in someone's home you have to be careful what you say and remember not to get comfortable with the family or the patient. Sometimes we are a go between because the spouse is abusive in one way or another.

They can always say they heard me wrong and you are not allowed to tape them or record them. So although you tell the proper authorities or your boss it sometimes falls on deaths ears.

You can and will get fired or taking off that assignment for wanting to do the right thing.

You see spouses or children yelling at their parents and telling them with all their PhDs look how you ended up not controlling your bladder and bowels. How the one you always favored is not here for you now.

What are you waiting for just die already. Children flying in only when they think that they are at deaths door and they bounce back and their off again you never see them.

It is sad but true but I see it all the time. Or people that cannot face the inevitable and blame it on everyone and God sue the facilities and anyone else they can think of.

You feel bad and want to help but it is sometimes hard to help an angry person that has their mind set. You can try avoiding them or say nothing.

Now the nursing homes have changed over the years it is not just elderly people it's all ages of people. That's why some of them had to change from old folks home to nursing home.

We have all sorts of patients from alcoholics to paraplegics.

In nursing we were never trained to take care of younger people Alzheimer's and dementia. Well if they have to train us how to take of young people and their mental state as a paraplegic. Drug addicts and how to counter act their behavior then they would have to pay us more money. Same treatment across the board.

Well I'm here to tell you that does not work. We had this young man of twenty six that was in a car accident that he caused. When he finally became coherent he was in a nursing home where nobody was there his own age or even close to it.

He didn't want to play bingo or have a sing along to the nineteen twenties. He got depressed and wanted out he left a few times but he found his old friends didn't want anything to do with him.

He came back and was told if he left for more than twenty four hours again he would lose his room.

Now Chris was racist and mean but he was twenty six. I waited one day I just wanted to talk to him offer him some hope and prayers he had to listen because he was in the bed and couldn't move , when he was in his chair I couldn't catch him.
He appeared to be happy getting better and use to his new normal.

I left for the week and came back he was dead, they said he took a bunch of pills and killed himself.

Pause, now he had barely functioning arms he needed help just to put his two fingers up to work his chair. I don't think he killed himself I think someone assisted with his suicide, but all speculation on my part.

Then there was my Jeremy that had all the hope in the world, had MS since he was twelve but believed in God and had a positive outlook. He actually was going to marry one of the nurses and have a kid. She was willing and wanted to take care of him.

Well other people didn't approve they thought it was disgusting. That a nurse fell in love with him, what was she doing when she was supposed to be working.

They fired her when he told them he was marrying her, didn't stop her from seeing him though he also was twenty six. One day someone had picked him up broke his hip he was dead in forty eight hours. A freak accident they called it.

There are people that stand out, that you just cannot forget and you often think to yourself what happened. You can't prove it because you weren't there and if you say anything your causing trouble.

Well these are people I have grown fond of knowing, they tell you their struggles and history piece by piece everyday as they are getting bathed or dressed or you just cleaned their room.

Again this is not furniture or appliances these are real live breathing, once had a life before the one you have come to see.

I stress this no matter what they deserve to go out with dignity and respect. It's hard sometimes I'm not going to lie. I have come to learn that even my worst patients have a story and that there is still a person behind that racist, mean, condescending always rude person.

You just have to look a little harder to find it and learn not to take it personal or learn the art of faking.

This young lady that a took care of her name was Dorothy she got Alzheimer's early and she was very aware of what was happening. She was a tough lady a woman foreman in a society that didn't believe in the equality of women.

She married her husband because that is what she was taught to do. However she had another plan let him teach me what he knows then I can become a boss one day.

Well she did just that and she had no children, just a niece she was fond of and helped raised her. Well as she noticed the development of the disease, she sold her house and checked herself in the nursing home. She didn't want to become a burden to anyone.
She often joked about it Kisha if I start to forget remind me.

One day my favorite lady got sick we did vitals they said it was the flu. Then I came back one day just to check on her and I thought it was pudding on her mouth but her lips where blue. She still had a pulse I yelled for the nurse and she called 911.

This is not a swanky well to do nursing home.

So the emt's come with and attitude and start arguing with the nurse. The start asking Dorothy some information but she is lethargic.

He says maybe she doesn't want to go to the hospital did you ask her. I finally screamed you assholes take her to the god damn hospital she is dying, my friend is dying.

The hospital was only five minutes away, she died in two days. Natural causes they said, her lips where blue with medicine she didn't swallow still in her mouth.

I always say what is on my mind, I try very hard to be respectful. It is hard when you no longer respect what you do. How this is the only thing you can see yourself doing that came natural since you were a kid. It is becoming shattered every day, with the lack of respect and honor it once had.

It is never how much you care or how long you have been there. It is how much they can get out of you until they can replace you. In every field we have learned as these years go on there is no such thing as irreplaceable.

Don't think I'm not going to name, names I am, just wait for it. I am going to name the death traps to the better ones even if they discriminate.

First I have to tell you about my friend yes there is more than I can tell which is sad again but true.

There was Donna angry at the world and had no particular person she just hated everyone. As I said it has always been my mission the harder they are, the more I want to help or find out why they are angry. I paid close attention to her what she ate and what she wasn't supposed to eat.

Like almost every diabetic they want what they can't have. She would go out with her wheelchair and go to the store across the street from the nursing home and buy ho hos and donuts.

Her favorite was Coca Cola. One day I decided to talk to her and ask this one legged, cursing everybody out maniac a simple question.

Would you like a Coke? Why she asked? Did you put something in it? Are you trying to bribe me to take my meds? No, I have nothing to do with your meds. It's getting cold, I'm not saying thank you she said. I said Ok.

Nothing else until she saw me again two days later. You have another coke you want to give away?

I can get one out the machine, I got some extra change. In the employees lounge the residents wasn't allowed in there.
There was no machine just my lunch box full of coke.

So I went to go get it and gave it to her. What do you want for it? "She said." I'll give you a coke a day if you tell no one and tell me one thing about yourself.

So she said she would but, I could tell she was hesitant. She asked me why are you being so nice and giving your cokes away to the one, I know they call a bitch.

Glutting for punishment I guess. So this went on for a month I would say. I would share Newport's with her and give her coke.
I don't smoke or drink coke. She started to tell me about herself, slowly.

She was born on my mother's birthday. She had a long time boyfriend that kicked her out as soon as her leg was amputated. Her father stopped speaking to her and her sister stopped coming to see her.

She was not without fault, she was angry and alienated everyone she just didn't know how to fix it.

She wore gloves because she had
neuropathy in her hands. She use to
ask me to text for her or open things
she couldn't. So I use to text her
family acting like a hard time with her
old flip phone.

I don't know if she knew to this day
that I called her dad and sister. It didn't
matter they started speaking to her
again.
The old boyfriend started coming to
see her and buying her things asking
for forgiveness.

Don't get me wrong she was still mean
as hell, she just wasn't mean to me all
the time or as rough. Over time she
wanted to walk again with a prosthetic.
I took a picture of her walking, I use to
encourage her that there was hope.

I use to talk to her allot I use to work 3-11 11-7 sixteen hour shifts on the weekend. In my down time I would talk to her she told me she was angry that the facility was getting the bulk her money and they got an allowance every month of about forty three dollars.

I did a little investigating, I mean she had her issues but she was only fifty she was just a diabetic. They did only give the residents that knew what was going on an allowance.

What did they do with the rest? From their disability checks after they got their share from the government. Remember 3,000 dollars a month or more per person from the government or private pay.

She wanted to challenge them and called a lawyer. These days the lawyers are all over cases from the nursing homes. She accused them of cheating her and she wanted more of her money.

They said she couldn't find a home on her on to take care of herself. She said she could use the disability money to find her own home.

People with disabilities live on their own every day. I thought she could do it. She showed me paper work of different agencies trying to reach her. However the facility said she was always unavailable. People with disabilities and Alzheimer's any debilitating disease is guaranteed money.

They sign all of these papers and talk
to so many people upon arrival,
usually they are still doped up from the
hospital stay or just plain out of it from
the shock of their present state. They'll
sign anything to get it over with and
these are trusted "nursing authorities".

You signed that you could not take
care of yourself. You don't remember
that though. Your signature, remember
ignorance of the law is no excuse for
its repercussions. Now what, you fight.

Well she all of a sudden got sick. I was
gone for the week but I always checked
up on her. I called she didn't answer. I
went up there, and she was in the bed
she just was starring off into space.

What's wrong with her? She stopped taking her meds. No, she wouldn't do that, she is enjoying life again. They took her out on stretcher, within a week she died from congested heart failure.

Every year I have a coke on her birthday and every time I see a truck I say hey Donna.

I'm not telling you these stories to horrify or bash the nursing field. Well maybe I am. You should be horrified and the powers that be should be ashamed of what they let the nursing field become.

Not only do the people deserve better that we take care of but we deserve better that take care of them. What I see doing survey time I want to see all the time. Everybody on the floor helping from top to bottom.

More variety of food, bonuses and special pay for the people that work hard. More variety of entertainment and activities for the young and the old.

More than one survey a year, more gratitude from your employer. No more people dying or getting hurt unnecessarily, people that meds for psych or behavioral matters.

Don't hide behind you shouldn't medicate people just to keep them quiet. No it's to keep them as sane as possible and us from getting abused unnecessarily.

Assess each patient it's not a one size fits all thing. We can't be everywhere at all times. One person to ten or twenty residents it's not humanly possible.

It they are falling constantly an alarm is not going to keep them from falling it just lets us know they fail.

Some restraints are necessary, yes it looks horrible but it does its job it stops them from falling.

Stop telling the family members that they can have what they want all the time to appease them. Have a backbone and tell them for the safety of your loved ones and the workers we must use the latest equipment.

Such as Hoyer lifts to prevent injury for both parties. No matter how big or small, heavy or light.

I am still using my back I would like to keep it thank you very much. Stop telling the patients they can abuse us and turn on the light for their anything they want.

We are there to help and do patient care, we are not the bell hops at a hotel. We are taking care of needs not egos. We are not there to relive roots.

Just because we chose this profession it does not mean we are stupid. If I am nursing assistant I maybe studying to be a L.P.N or not. Just because I have an accent it doesn't mean I don't speak English.

To people that speak other languages and are from somewhere else, you talk funny to and they always understand you.

Just because I am a L.P.N. the joke is not funny that I am just practicing and I am not a real nurse. School is hard and grueling and I had to take the state boards. So fuck you I earned this.

Doctors I am your ears and back bone, I see what you didn't catch because you were in a rush or you were just tired. I am an R.N. stop giving me your mightier than thou superiority God complex shit.

Stop telling us that you can take someone from McDonald's and train them to do this work. While that may be true, they don't have the stomach for it. Guess what they have better benefits and make more money. So what does that say about your devalue of us.

We understand that this is a business, but stop treating it like it's an assembly line. You own it but next to never step foot in it. We are dealing with people and lives that matter.

Remember I am calling you out "Nursing" get back to the people and the matter of caring about both sides.

Now for that list as promised now I don't or didn't work at all of these but we in Nursing talk to each other.

Now for legal purposes I can't put the Exact names but I will not leave it to your imagination I promise.

If you want your family member to die a quick or slow painful death,you will take them to Coso Mora of Bradenton Florida. Bradeen River of Bradenton. Rivera Palms of Palmetto Florida. Accenti in Tampa discriminates and if you don't fall in to their money category you can't get in.
West or east Minister Towers tells their employees that it doesn't matter how many residents they have, that you are paid slaves. Palm Rive,Heritag park,Herwthorne Village.

Now usually the nursing homes that are for profit only are the worst, they treat their employees like shit and the residents they give two cents about. They call are make a fuss when they see their money is being spent or it seems its being given away, God forbid they pay you for one extra minute.

The nursing homes that a non profit they are usually the best to work for, the best pay and they actually care. Yes they are getting paid but they take care of their employees and residents much more pleasant environment and better everything from food to supplies.

Anything owned by St. Josephs Fantastic. Sarasota of Pines they are struggling a little bit now because of new management but I am confident that they will get back on track.

Sarasota Jewish Community takes great care of their residents and employees. Even though it is a for profit company it has been in business for many years passed down from generations. They make it a point to take of their employees and the residents they understand that happy employees means happy residents. Overall moral is high because of something so simple they value you and they make it a point to tell you often.

Yeah whatever the pay should be its own reward is a crock. I want you to show me and tell me that this would not work without you and mean it. I'm not saying lie to me as we have learned. If I'm doing a bad job tell me so I can improve but also if I'm doing a great job tell me.

Now I also understand with reading this book that people may think I am just a disgruntle employee. No it's quite the opposite I can work anywhere but my conscious of that fifteen year old girl won't let me. I have been fired but I don't hold grudges. I just want to see nursing get back to basics.

The truth is even though it is our worst fear people in nursing that is. Young or old you can wind up in a place like this and you want to know that the person taking care of you has the basic understanding of compassion and common decency. Your life and well being could be in hands of these healthcare professionals. Let us get back to treating each other with dignity and respect.

Or again learn the art of faking.

About the Author: I Kisha Brown age 45 Three Children four grandchildren Two sisters and two brothers and two very supportive parents have been in nursing for twenty years. It has put food on the table. I was fifteen years old when I decided I was either going to be a person that worked in a graveyard or in a hospital. Morbid but true somebody is always sick and somebody is always dying. Well I didn't know I would feel such a sense of pride other than raising my kids. People that needed me sounded like a great profession. I have been happy for the most part to be a Nursing Assistant.